Best Selling Author Dr. Sophia Edwards-Bennett Presents

HIGHER GROUND

THE TRANSFORMATIVE POWER OF THE BIG-C (CANCER) RE-ATTITUDES

Sophia Edwards-Bennett
Tampa, FL, USA
Mydoctoreb.com

Ordering Information:
For details, contact: MyDoctorEB@gmail.com

Print ISBN: 978-1-7373151-0-0

Printed in the United States of America on SFI Certified paper.

First Edition

Preface

Recently, I was blessed with the opportunity to be a coauthor with Jack Canfield and other thought leaders in the book *Success*.

However, my chapter entitled *Higher Ground*, did not provide steps or a blueprint to success.
Instead, I wrote about the peri-center of my fulfillment, a subject of moments of cerebral saturation.
Because, that is my definition of success: fulfillment, gained from dedicating your time and energy to a career that is also a life passion.
For me, that is medicine, specifically oncology.
Beyond a shadow of doubt, I was divinely ordained to serve, to help, and to heal cancer patients.

To serve, by not just being the cancer doctor with the expertise, awards and accolades. But one that is thoughtfully conceptualizing, crafting and drafting unchartered methods.

To not singularly focus on treating the cancer.
But to also target the often ignored, but significant, casualties of the diagnosis of cancer: the psychological lacerations, the emotional infections, the mental abscess, the threatening hopelessness, the taunting fears and soundtrack of plaguing anxieties; the sequelae of life after the diagnosis, that certainly do not end with their cancer treatment course.

To guide cancer patients through this very dauntingly difficult process, I must equip my patients with a sound and comprehensive tool box; an armamentarium for the life they did not choose, that was beyond their control.

To accomplish this, a transformation of the mind lies at the foundation. Providing an armor, a shield, a helmet, and a sword for their new lives' journey.
Hope, Identity, Self-Worth/Esteem, Life Appraisal, Admiration Requited, Mind Rehabilitation and Purpose.

These are the core elements of their PPE (P*ersonal Protective Equipmen*t), the essential components of **The Big C Re-Attitudes.**

So, that was my focus in the book *Success.*
A tad unorthodox, I know....
But I was indeed honored to contribute to that body of work.

However, for my patient's sake, and for their loved ones, caretakers, and also other like-minded oncologists; I thought it was important to assign/ascribe it, its own entity. To portray and provide a short, clear, directly accessible algorithm, a practical guide for facile, clinical implementation.

In this book, I have also included commentaries, bonus proses, and *a chant for my cancer patients*. The latter, I hope will become an inspirational *anthem of sorts*, for cancer patients around the globe.

I created the audio version, so that when you listen, you will know, that although the voice speaks, the heart is the true source.

So, from my heart to yours.

Sincerely,

Sophia Edwards-Bennett

Dr. EB

Best Selling Author Dr. Sophia Edwards-Bennett Presents

HIGHER GROUND

THE TRANSFORMATIVE POWER OF THE BIG-C (CANCER) RE-ATTITUDES

CONTENTS

Introduction of the Author

First, allow me to introduce myself
I'm Dr. Sophia Edwards-Bennett, aka Dr EB,
That's what all my patients and colleagues call me
To which, I have conceded
To the thousands of cancer patients I've been honored to have met and treated

Here's what I want you to know, undoubtedly

Whether or not we have met personally
Our spirits connect in some dimension
And in that realm, I hope that this book invokes within you, a familiar emotion

I share this with you , with all its prose
To render insight , composed, written
Not focused on cancer only, but in fact, in lieu
To shine the light on simply you
To unveil the unique essence that you imbue
So that you , *YES YOU*, will be revealed to you too...

So, from all those who love you so very dearly
Through distance, space and time
Hearts and minds virtually, collectively intertwined

Read on and you'll see
That, we all unanimously agree

It is absolutely, most genuinely true
We are.......

Sincerely,
Thinking of you

Commentary

Welcome to the audible of the book *Success, Chapter 10*, entitled '***Higher Ground'***, by me: Sophia Edwards-Bennett MD., PhD, aka Dr. EB.

Allow me to render the commentary, a bonus, as promised and advertised.

Success can be defined as, characterized by, or ascribed to, multiple different outcomes.

However, I define success as fulfilling one's purpose.
I must state, that I am indeed blessed to be endowed with the gifts, to fulfill my calling; which is to serve my patients in the capacity of a Radiation Oncologist.

It is this sense of true purpose which spawned my passion; to do more, to see more, and to be more, for my patients.
And in return, my patients not only entrust me with their lives, but they invite me into their minds, bear their souls, and reveal their spirits.

My *purposed passion, coupled with their naked souls,* seeds my desire and fuels the mental sojourn for a remedy, a method, an antidote that goes beyond the cancer; to arrest their fears and anxieties; that constellation of physiological toxicities that inevitably results from facing one's mortality.

And so, from this, the **Big C Re: Attitudes** was borne-which I highlight in this chapter.

A 7 -pronged approach, to not only help patients cope with the psychological toxicities; but to overcome them, refine their emotional dexterity, and sharpen their mental fortitude.

The Big C Re-Attitudes, as you will discover herein, address *Hope, Identity, Self-worth/esteem, Life appraisal, Admiration /Affirmation,*

Mind Rehabilitation and Renewed Purpose.

So, in summary, the success of my patients' healing, is gained from my success, which is the fulfillment of my purpose.

HIGHER GROUND

BY SOPHIA EDWARDS-BENNETT, M.D., Ph.D., DABR

[Dedication: To the Author and Finisher of our Faith.]

The Transformative Power of the Big-C (Cancer) Re-Attitudes

I once climbed Blue Mountain in Jamaica with a group of friends. A grand idea at the time, mystical even, laced with florid thoughts of bonding with friends, sharing, and cheering. And all that was true, but the hike was grueling, arduous, and much longer than I envisioned; not infrequently plagued with thoughts of quitting, alternating with self-probing questions about the impetus for my initial commitment to this venture.

But the travail was all anesthetized upon our arrival at the summit; at the cool of 5:45 am, with fresh June air whisking gently across my face as I stood, in the ensuing moments, catatonic, gasping at the emerging stunning sunrise.

I expanded the ambit of my circumferential gaze to the captivating panoramic view, and the incredible aerial landscape below.

I stood still, aware of every heartbeat, every breath, inhaling the sheer awe of it all.
The view from above, an unassailable canvas of creation's wonder.

And there it was, a new perspective, while standing on *higher ground.*

I submit that there is a parallel metaphorical correlate of life, that is, *a higher ground*, preceded by seemingly insurmountable obstacles, challenges that inevitably conjure thoughts of doubt, and deposit seeds of fear.

But with perquisite marination in time, it unleashes our innate tenacity, resilience, endurance, and fortitude of the mind; providing the essential coordinates to navigate our route to '*higher ground.*'

It is from that vantage, that one's perspective is ideally perched – to transcend the metaphysical gamut, gleaning a higher order of perception, of unchartered dimensions.

The question is:

How do we attain that higher dimension that liberates our minds? How do we gain enlightenment that lends copious insight, adorning us with wings of faith?

The answer is, quite complex, variegated with critique
As, our inner battles are both personal and unique.

Our revelations, synthesized by our innermost truths
Are our very own customized stories.
Colored by our experiences and primed by our roots.

PRELUDE

My Serum of Truth
A higher ground-I believe, is where success is found
Carving a path where tales of my destiny abound
Epiphanies gleaned from a coalescence of vicissitudinous waves.
Revelations from the oxymorons of life
Lends itself to the first of a series of: *Prose for Ponder*

The meat of the matter: Revelations from the oxymorons of our lives

It's not monolithic, but amorphous
It's not defined, but irregular and unpredictable
It's not ubiquitously applied but uniquely ascribed
But it is including, but not limited to,
The amalgamation of experiential encounters,
The exhilarating and the devastating
The soulful good and the indiscriminate evil
The inexplicable adversarial and the welcomed collegial
Our failures and fecundities
The terrains of tears and the fallacy of our fears
The veracity in our vulnerability and the nescience of our naivety
The hives of hypocrisy and the hailing of honesty
The truce of trust and the poise of peace
These collective experiences amassed...
Our reflexive reactions, ensued by reflections upon,
and revelations thereof...
The analytic appraisals and granular interpretations
They infiltrate our inchoate beings, exquisitely and meticulously mold us
And inform our evolutionary transformation to becoming
Until we indeed become...
The true and best version of ourselves.
That's the meat ...of the matter.... of our lives.

The Real Heroes: Chronicles of the Cancer Patient

Whenever I meet people in any setting, professional or otherwise
Questions prompt my disclosure that I'm an oncologist.
To which a frequent reaction is— 'that must be really tough!'
And while it is undeniably difficult, it is also indubitably rewarding.
But my experience pales in comparison to the overwhelming, indescribable, adverse challenges faced by cancer patients.

I often espouse the statement that my patients are my teachers, heroes indeed; with a remarkable display of courage and candor, an irrefutable truth to which we all magnanimously concede.

CHRONICLES OF THE CANCER PATIENT

Insight on Invasion
Through my lens, from their eyes

Imagine going about your normal daily lives.
Interacting with family, friends, and the occasional stranger
Enacting responsibilities at work and home.
Making plans for the future as we all do; vacations, family traditions, milestone events such as anniversaries and birthdays and other recurring social events.

Then one day you notice, perchance, a hard area in the breast, a lingering headache unlike your occasional tension headache, lasting longer than usual; an uncharacteristic cough, or inexplicable weight loss that you've craved for in the past, but at this juncture is suspiciously effortless.

Your initial reaction is to bury these cryptic feelings of uncertainty, the discomfort of uneasiness.
But the nagging feelings re-emerge, as the growing knot in your stomach wounds tighter by the second.
So finally, you cajole yourself to see your primary doctor.

Now, let's fast forward to the moment of truth.
After multiple probing tests have been performed…
Your doctor walks in the room, wearing a solemn face.
A tell-tale sign of bad news.

And, as you hear the word *CANCER, the BIG-C*
Time seems to stand still….
As you 'subconsciously' dissociate from yourself
And you find yourself in the weird unchartered space of feeling 'outside of yourself'.

You observe yourself from a distance, through blurred lenses,

Listening to the now seemingly distant voice of your doctor describing factoids,
And the myriad of recommended treatments you'll have to endure.

<u>Prose for Ponder</u>

You listen with pause
With wandering mind
Willing yourself to hear the details
Some bold and verbally <u>underlined</u>
While others are italicized
Another treatment, another phase, another odyssey in kind

Overwhelmed, I listen carefully, in this decorated room with ambient light,
Translation, another battle in this life to fight.

And you ask yourself ….
Is this really happening to me?

This psychological spiraling can be devastating and paralyzing.

The reaction I've described above, is certainly within the realm of a normal human reaction.
Understandably so as, after all, facing one's mortality is one of life's greatest fears.
And even after successful treatment, cancer patients are perpetually plagued with the fear of recurrence.

This psychological aftermath can be debilitating, so much so that their sense of self, life, its value and purpose, is trapped in a somber cycle.

Perseveration and rumination becoming their *modus vivendi*: their way of life
As it consumes their thoughts.

Wishing it was just a nightmare, rising each morning to the rude awakening that it's not a dream, but in actuality, their reality.

Prose for Ponder

Lonely with my tears I lie….
With not a morsel f energy left to cry
Restless and confused
But most of all, my life I'm scared to lose
A dream I hope from which I'll awake.
Then perils I see, will disappear for my sanity's sake
But alas, I open my eyes and find familiar space
As the flicker of light sneaks through the curtains and shines on my face
It's true, it's happening and it's real.
Cancer is the diagnosis, and there is no appeal.

This psychologically-debilitating stampede is concerning; but even more disturbing is the fact that several studies have demonstrated that patients' psychological status impacts their actual quality of life.

Now, due to the heterogeneous nature of the methods used to address the psychological needs of cancer patients, metanalyses of these studies (grouping the results of multiple studies to generate a larger number of cases and thus more reliable results) have demonstrated varying outcomes.[1,2] However, the effect on patients' quality of life remains consistent.

But sadly, many patients do not seek psychological counsel, which is consequentially detrimental to their quality of life.

One might ask, why?
Why don't patients seek psychological counsel?

The most common reasons are the diagnoses, required treatment schedule, and management of side effects are overwhelming and time-consuming, thus precluding the procurement of psychological counsel; or reticence to seek counsel due to the stigma attached to the admission of the need for psychological intervention, or the unwillingness to endorse the need for any help at all, fueled by the need to portray and evince, strength and independence.

When patients present to me, they expect treatment for cancer. And that I do, employing all the knowledge and experience in my armamentarium. This approach, albeit dutiful and commendable, does not guarantee access to the psychological landscape of my patients.

As an oncologist, I recognize that my patients are entrusting me with their most precious gift—their lives.

It is within this contextual construct that I believe that I am uniquely positioned to not only provide them with the best possible cancer treatment, but also play an integral role in reshaping their psychological frame of mind.

I do so by invoking what I have coined, the **Big-C Re-Attitudes**: to enlighten and empower patients to cope with their diagnosis, treatment and beyond.

These **Re-Attitudes** include:

- **Re**appraisal of Life
- **Re**storation of Hope
- **Re**clamation of Identity
- **Re**affirmation of Self-Worth
- **Re**habilitation of the Mind
- **Re**ignition of Purpose
- **Re**quited Admiration

How is this invocation accomplished?

Just as cancer treatment needs to be tailored to the stage and other unique features of a patient's cancer, a customized approach must be ascribed to address each patient's psychological blueprint.

But to construct, I must first deconstruct, to expose the warfare in the mind, frequently expressed solely by inner screams and outward silence.

To do this effectively, it is imperative that I develop a solid relationship with my patients, to inspire trust and elicit vulnerability. I do this by employing a customized, multistep interactive process, commencing from the time of consultation, progressing through treatment and beyond, to follow-up after treatment.

It is during these encounters that I observe, listen, and ascertain information, from which I can then formulate a custom-made strategy for each patient, to effectively infuse **The Big-C Re-Attitudes**.

These *Big-C Re-attitudes* are borne out of the exploration of several important, probing questions. The probing questions are directed toward my patients and me.

Yes indeed, the formulation of the *Big-C Re-Attitudes* requires my equal participation. This reciprocity evokes vulnerability and endears trust.

What are these probing questions?
I'll highlight a few.....

1) What do you most treasure or enjoy about life?
2) What qualities do patients emanate; in other words, what unique attributes do I discern in my patients, that can be augmented and refocused toward their own psychological development?
3) What lessons does each patient teach those they encounter?
4) How have these lessons learned contributed to the enrichment of the lives of patients' family, friends, and other close encounters?

Information gleaned from these questions, yields a new narrative that I can utilize to inform and construct a customized set of **Big-C Re-Attitudes** for each patient.

So, in effect, I 'plant the seeds' to eventually harvest The Big-C Re-Attitudes.

These attributes, although closely intertwined, must be unearthed by the execution of a systematic, methodical, ardent and sequential process, with measured sedimentation and filtering, given the complex psychological state of a cancer patient.

However, the results yield a defined tool-set, designed to be applied in their daily lives, transforming their minds to create healthier psychological beings.

A truly remarkable dividend, is that upon the repetitive application of this algorithm, cancer patients are also uniquely positioned, having experienced its transmuting effects, to authentically disseminate the 'gospel' of the *Big-C Re-Attitudes*, by imparting their 'serum of truth'.

An even more auspicious prospect is, that upon propagation by, and to other, cancer patients, the baton can be relayed to friends and colleagues, whose lives have also been directly or indirectly affected by cancer, resulting in a ripple effect. Simply remarkable.

Prose for Ponder

Restoration of Hope

This battle of hope
Is riddled with uncertainty
It's the life unknown
The one we dare, while the failures we fear
The dreaded days we face
While anticipated ones we embrace
It's the joys we treasure
With all the struggles unmeasured
But with armors of love, swords of truth
Inner strength and minds astute
Giving up, we ebulliently refuse

We have but one life, and it's ours to lose,
So we're ready for battle, hence, victory we will choose.

Prose for Ponder

***Re**clamation of Identity*

It's not the 'you' that they think they see
It's not the person they believe they perceive
But it's the real core of you, that you know holds true
That echoes in the words you say, and reflects in the deeds you do.

Prose for Ponder

***Re**affirmation of Self-Worth*

***Re**habilitation of the Mind*

In me, but not of me
It is the unwelcomed invader, I see
Threatening to cocoon the force I'm meant to be But I
will spout my manifold truth
After all, this is my story, to boot So I
will not stay silent
I refuse to be mute

Prose for ponder

***Re**appraisal of Life*

***Re**ignition of Purpose*

'Tis from the arduous journey That a
litany of experiences unfold
Composing a story that is destined to be told
That grief not wasted is happiness consulted
Doubt abated is conviction unscathed

Loss endured is gain secured Hope unaborted is faith consorted....
And adversity repealed is strength revealed.

PRE-EPILOGUE

We all desire a cure, the panacea for cancer.
But in the meantime, we can all play a role in enriching cancer patients' lives.

Of course, there is always a resistant force to any positive endeavor But, if we remain persuaded, if we are tenacious, intentional, and vigilant in executing our vision, we can all be beacons of light, transcendent of policies and protocols, honoring only the propagation of the seeds of hope, health, and life.

I am eager to share this transformative algorithm, The **Big-C Re-Attitudes**, which, based on my clinical experience, will significantly impact the psychological frame of mind of cancer patients, improving their quality of life and transforming their lives.

I also strongly believe that the institution and practice of the **Big-C Re-Attitudes** will inevitably improve the cancer patient-doctor relationship.

EPILOGUE

Last, not least……
Our patients effusively express their appreciation to us
Which I usually graciously accept.
But forthwith I pose this question—an idiomatic citation:

DO YOU SEE WHAT I SEE?

The answer underscores our *Requited Admiration* for our cancer patients:

While we treat them, they enlighten us
While we encourage them, they inspire us.

While we advise them, they edify us.
While we heal their bodies, they enrich our souls.

Because their journey embodies the resilience of humanity
Epitomizes the essence of hope and encapsulates the true
meaning of life.

Join me in sharing this transformative algorithm with the world
So that we can expand this vision of 'Saving lives while
transforming minds.'

...And collectively aspire to ***Higher Ground.***

"For with Him, all things are possible."

Appendix

Acronym for The Big-C Re-Attitudes

HIS LAMP

*Hope Identity Self-Worth Life Admiration Mind Purpose "**His** word is a **lamp** unto our feet, and a light unto our paths."*

References

1. Guarino A., Polini C., Forte G., Favieri F., Boncompagni I., and Casagrande,
M. **The Effectivenessof Psychological Treatmentsin Womenwith Breast Cancer: A Systematic Review and Meta-Analysis**. J Clin Med. 2020 Jan; 9(1): 209.

Myrhaug H.T., Mbalilaki J.A., Lie N.K., Hansen T., and Nordvik J.E. **The effects of multidisciplinary psychosocial interventions on adult cancer patients: A systematic review and meta-analysis**. Disabil. Rehabil. 2018:1–9.

Dr. EB Answers the Question Why?

Dr. EB answers the question: Why is it Important that the **Big C Re-Attitudes** be Instituted at the inception of diagnosis and treatment?

Why is this important?

This is a truly relevant and certainly pertinent question.

It is of paramount importance to intercede and infuse the **Big C Re-Attitudes** at the onset of diagnosis and treatment.
Because, you see once a seed is planted in the mental/psychological soil ....so to speak ...

Time then enables the corrosion of the mind.
It festers, reproducing and replicating anxiety and fear.
And this serves as a catalyst for the insurgence of the mind's stability, incarcerating the mind, emaciating self-esteem, and depleting hope.

But, when the **Big C Re-Attitudes** are instituted at the onset, then when patients are faced with the aftermath and unease about recurrence, or spread of disease that can ensue treatment; they are better equipped with all the acumens, the blueprint of the **Big C Re-Attitudes.**
Thus, providing a restructured framework, with an inventory of mental fortitude, emotional dexterity, and the psychological bandwidth to cope with the siege of worry than can ensue treatment.
So that., their 're-entrance' into the world so to speak, will be bolstered with, and anchored by, the **Big C Re-Attitudes.**

The Bridge

What is a bridge?

A bridge serves to connect people, places, and spaces.
It protects from, while preserving, what lies beneath it.

Its goal is to provide a secure passage.
By offering a path to be traversed
Irrespective of identity, hues and shades, language, culture, socioeconomic backgrounds, or creed.

The audiobook is presented as a bridge
A bridge of understanding for patients and physicians, loved ones, families and friend, acquaintances, and establishments.

And for every person, institution, or any entity, desiring a lucid, a clear understanding of our cancer patients' journey.
So that we can all be ...*The Bridge*

Now here is...A Chant for Cancer Patients

A Chant for Cancer Patients

You weren't invited
But you entered still
Against my will

And now you're here
To conjure fear

My heart to smear
My hope to dare

But I will fight
With all my might

I won't give up
I won't give in

Each I day I live
The battle I win
The battle I win
The battle I win

So I'll hold my kin
Closer and closer
My family, friends
I treasure hence....

I treasure hence
I'm not alone
I'm not alone
Through moans and groan

So It's not in vain
Through all the pain
More strength I gain
As I praise His name

HIGHER GROUND

I won't give up
I won't give in
Each I day I live
The battle I win

So I'll hold my kin
Closer and closer
My family, friends
I treasure hence..

I won't give up
I won't give in
Each I day I live
The battle I win

So it's not in vain
Through all the pain
More strength I gain
As I praise His name

Thank you

To you, *Yes You*, listening attentively
Wherever you are, or choose to be geographically
Or your state sublimed psychologically

You heeded the interest that you have harbored in your mind
You listened, expending your energy, and committing your time
For the sake of your fellow human in kind

To understand the depth, the breadth, of a cancer patient's journey

So, I am sure that I speak for us all
When I say most wholeheartedly
Thank you for heeding the call

The End!

Made in the USA
Monee, IL
04 November 2026

67386425R10020